AFIB DIET RECIPES COOKBOOK

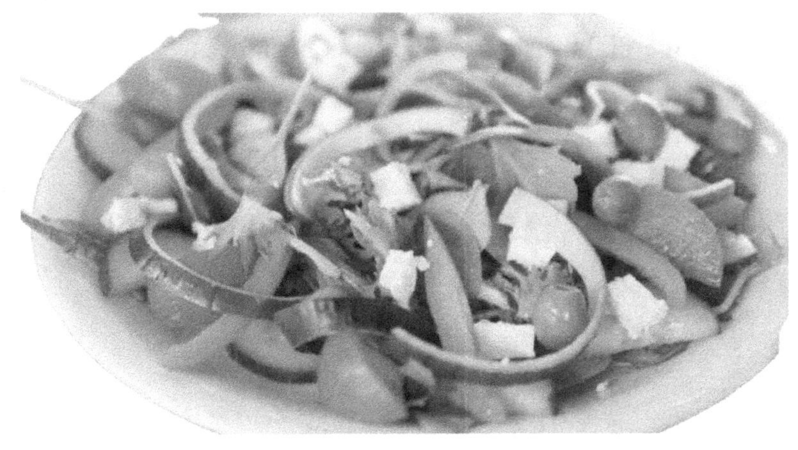

Dr. Kimberly Carlos

Copyright © 2023 by Dr. Kimberly Carlos

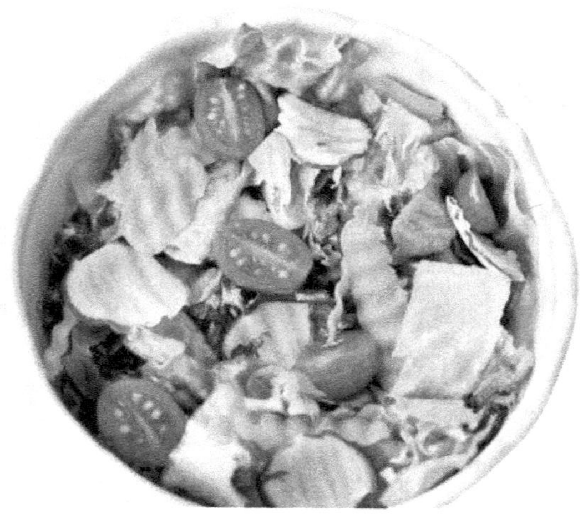

TABLE OF CONTENT

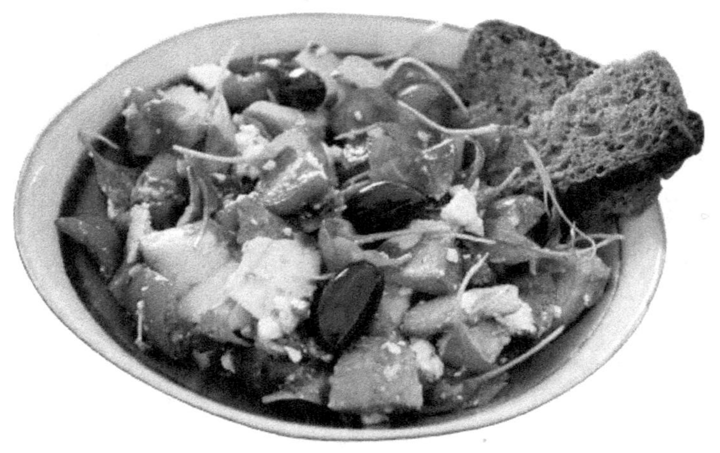

INTRODUCTION

Once upon a time, in a quaint village nestled between rolling hills, lived a man named Oliver. Oliver was known for his unbridled love for adventure, but his life took an unexpected turn when he was diagnosed with atrial fibrillation (AFib), a heart condition that left him feeling sluggish and apprehensive.

Determined not to let his condition define him, Oliver embarked on a journey of discovery. He stumbled upon a collection of AFib diet recipes - a treasure trove of dishes designed to support heart health.

With newfound determination, he began experimenting in his small kitchen, swapping out unhealthy ingredients for wholesome alternatives.

Oliver's mornings began with a vibrant berry and oat smoothie that kicked off his day with a burst of antioxidants and fiber. For lunch, he relished a colorful spinach and salmon salad, packed with omega-3 fatty acids that were said to promote heart health. But it was dinner that truly became his culinary canvas.

He crafted flavorful quinoa-stuffed bell peppers, roasted to perfection and brimming with a mix of veggies and lean protein.

As weeks turned into months, Oliver's energy began to rebound. He found himself less fatigued and more spirited, eager to tackle the outdoors once more. He went on gentle hikes, rekindling his love for nature, and made new friends in local support groups who shared his journey.

The village began to notice Oliver's transformation. Neighbors whispered about his renewed vigor, attributing it to his dedication to the AFib diet recipes. Soon, Oliver started hosting cooking workshops, sharing his culinary creations and knowledge with others who faced similar challenges. The aroma of wholesome meals filled the village, and a sense of community blossomed around heart-healthy living.

Oliver's journey not only revitalized his own life but touched the lives of many around him. He showed that with determination, a sprinkle of creativity, and a dash of heart-healthy ingredients, anyone could transform their fate. And so, his village learned that even in the face of adversity, a recipe for a better life was always within reach.

CHAPTER ONE

Afib Diet and Its Benefits

Atrial fibrillation (AFib) is a common heart rhythm disorder that affects millions of people around the world. While medical treatments play a crucial role in managing AFib, adopting a heart-healthy diet can significantly contribute to better management and improved quality of life.

In this book, we'll delve into the details of following an AFib diet, exploring its benefits and providing practical tips for integrating these dietary changes into your life.

Understanding the AFib Diet

The AFib diet focuses on making informed food choices that support heart health and help manage the condition's symptoms. It emphasizes nutrient-rich foods while minimizing those that may trigger AFib episodes or exacerbate its effects. Key elements of the AFib diet include:

1. Balanced Nutrition: Prioritize a diet rich in whole foods, including fruits, vegetables, whole grains, lean proteins, and healthy fats. These provide essential vitamins, minerals, and antioxidants that help maintain heart health.

2. Low Sodium Intake: Reducing sodium intake helps manage blood pressure, a crucial factor in managing AFib. Opt for fresh foods and limit processed and packaged foods, which are often high in sodium.

3. Healthy Fats: Incorporate sources of healthy fats, such as avocados, nuts, seeds, and fatty fish like salmon, which provide omega-3 fatty acids that support heart health and reduce inflammation.

4. Limit Caffeine and Alcohol: Excessive caffeine and alcohol consumption can trigger AFib episodes in some individuals. Moderation is key, and you might consider eliminating or reducing these substances if they seem to impact your condition.

5. Magnesium and Potassium: Foods rich in magnesium and potassium, such as leafy greens, bananas, and beans, can help maintain proper heart rhythm and muscle function.

Benefits of Following an AFib Diet

1. Improved Heart Health: The primary benefit of the AFib diet is its positive impact on heart health. Nutrient-dense foods can support cardiovascular function, reduce inflammation, and lower the risk of developing other heart-related complications.

2. Stabilized Blood Pressure: A diet low in sodium and rich in potassium can help regulate blood pressure, reducing strain on the heart and decreasing the risk of AFib episodes.

3. Reduced Inflammation: Chronic inflammation is linked to heart disease and AFib. An AFib diet rich in antioxidants and anti-inflammatory compounds can mitigate inflammation, potentially reducing the frequency and severity of AFib episodes.

4. Weight Management: Adopting an AFib diet can contribute to weight management or weight loss, which is particularly beneficial for those with AFib. Maintaining a healthy weight reduces the risk of complications and improves overall heart function.

5. Enhanced Energy Levels: Nutrient-dense foods provide sustained energy throughout the day, combating fatigue and enhancing your ability to engage in physical activity.

Practical Tips for Following an AFib Diet

1. Consult a Healthcare Professional: Before making any significant dietary changes, consult your healthcare provider, especially if you are on medication. They can provide personalized guidance based on your medical history and needs.

2. Keep a Food Diary: Track your meals and any symptoms you experience. This can help you identify potential triggers and assess the effectiveness of your dietary changes.

3. Plan Balanced Meals: Create well-rounded meals that incorporate a variety of nutrient-rich foods. Aim for a balance of carbohydrates, proteins, and healthy fats.

4. Read Labels: Pay attention to nutritional labels to identify sodium content in packaged foods. Choose low-sodium or sodium-free options whenever possible.

5. Stay Hydrated: Drink plenty of water to maintain hydration, support proper heart function, and aid digestion.

6. Choose Whole Grains: Opt for whole grains like quinoa, brown rice, and whole wheat over refined grains to provide sustained energy and essential nutrients.

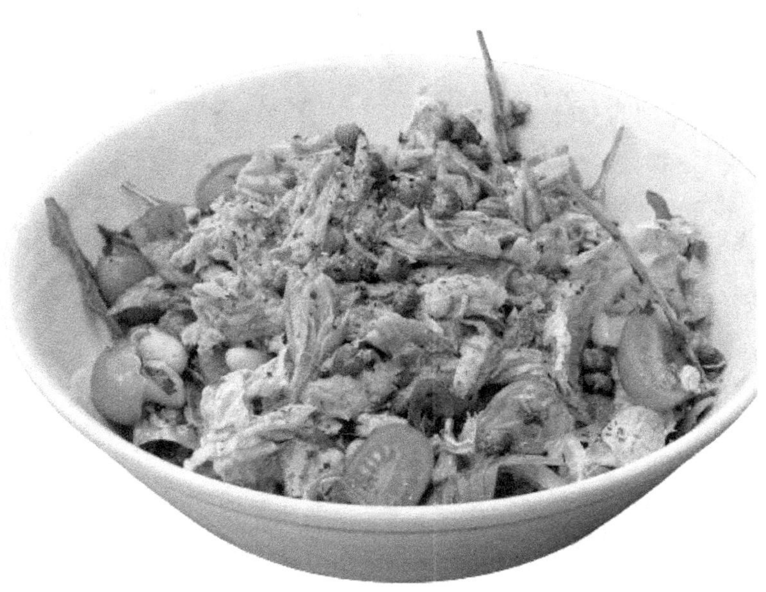

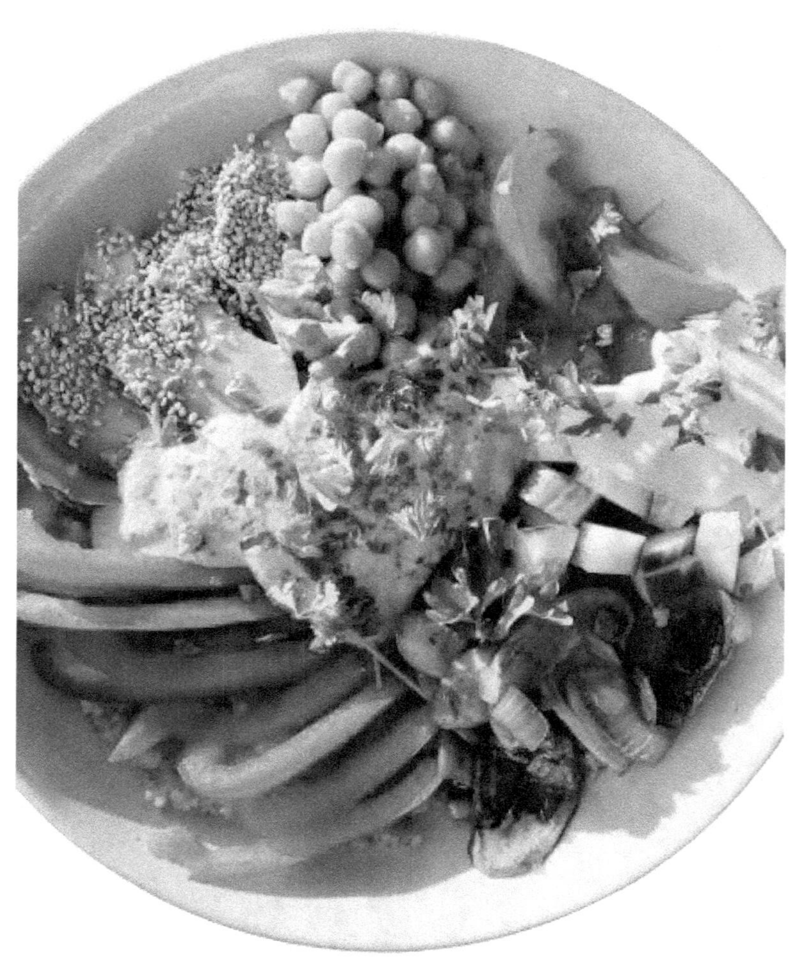

CHAPTER TWO

14-Day AFib Diet Meal Plan

Day 1

- **Breakfast:**
- Berry and Spinach Smoothie: Blend spinach, mixed berries, banana, chia seeds, almond milk, and a scoop of protein powder.
- **Lunch:**
- Grilled Chicken Salad: Mix grilled chicken, mixed greens, cucumber, bell peppers, cherry tomatoes, and a light vinaigrette dressing.
- **Dinner:**
- Baked Salmon: Serve with quinoa and steamed broccoli. Drizzle with lemon juice.

Day 2

- **Breakfast:**
- Greek Yogurt Parfait: Layer Greek yogurt, granola, mixed berries, and a drizzle of honey.
- **Lunch:**
- Chickpea and Avocado Salad: Combine chickpeas, avocado, red onion, cilantro, lime juice, and a sprinkle of feta cheese.
- **Dinner:**
- Turkey Meatballs: Serve with whole wheat pasta and a side of sautéed spinach.

Day 3

- **Breakfast:**
- Oatmeal with Almonds and Berries: Top cooked oats with chopped almonds, blueberries, and a dash of cinnamon.
- **Lunch:**
- Quinoa and Black Bean Bowl: Mix cooked quinoa, black beans, corn, diced bell peppers, and a lime-cilantro dressing.
- **Dinner:**
- Grilled Veggie Stir-Fry: Combine a variety of colorful vegetables with tofu or lean protein. Serve over brown rice.

Day 4

- **Breakfast:**
- Whole Wheat Toast with Avocado: Spread avocado on whole wheat toast and sprinkle with red pepper flakes.
- **Lunch:**
- Lentil and Vegetable Soup: Prepare a hearty soup with lentils, carrots, celery, onions, and low-sodium vegetable broth.

- **Dinner:**
- Lemon Herb Roasted Chicken: Pair with roasted sweet potatoes and steamed asparagus.

Day 5

- **Breakfast:**
- Smoothie Bowl: Blend frozen banana, spinach, almond milk, and a scoop of protein powder. Top with sliced almonds and fresh fruit.
- **Lunch:**
- Tuna Salad Lettuce Wraps: Mix canned tuna, diced celery, red onion, and light mayo. Wrap in lettuce leaves.
- **Dinner:**
- Grilled Vegetable and Quinoa Stuffed Bell Peppers: Serve with a side salad.

Day 6

- **Breakfast:**
- Scrambled Eggs with Veggies: Sauté bell peppers, onions, and spinach. Mix with scrambled eggs and a sprinkle of low-fat cheese.
- **Lunch:**
- Hummus and Veggie Wrap: Spread hummus on a whole wheat tortilla, add sliced cucumber, shredded carrots, and baby spinach.

- **Dinner:**
- Baked Cod: Serve with roasted Brussels sprouts and a quinoa salad with cherry tomatoes and parsley.

Day 7

- **Breakfast:**
- Chia Seed Pudding: Combine chia seeds, almond milk, vanilla extract, and a touch of honey. Refrigerate overnight and top with mixed berries.
- **Lunch:**
- Roasted Vegetable Quinoa Bowl: Mix roasted vegetables, cooked quinoa, and a drizzle of balsamic vinaigrette.
- **Dinner:**
- Grilled Portobello Mushrooms: Serve as "burgers" on whole wheat buns, with a side of grilled zucchini.

Day 8

- **Breakfast:**
- Berry and Spinach Smoothie: Blend spinach, mixed berries, banana, chia seeds, almond milk, and a scoop of protein powder.
- **Lunch:**
- Grilled Chicken Salad: Mix grilled chicken, mixed greens, cucumber, bell peppers, cherry tomatoes, and

a light vinaigrette dressing.
- **Dinner:**
- Baked Salmon: Serve with quinoa and steamed broccoli. Drizzle with lemon juice.

Day 9

- **Breakfast:**
- Greek Yogurt Parfait: Layer Greek yogurt, granola, mixed berries, and a drizzle of honey.
- **Lunch:**
- Chickpea and Avocado Salad: Combine chickpeas, avocado, red onion, cilantro, lime juice, and a sprinkle of feta cheese.
- **Dinner:**
- Turkey Meatballs: Serve with whole wheat pasta and a side of sautéed spinach.

Day 10

- **Breakfast:**
- Oatmeal with Almonds and Berries: Top cooked oats with chopped almonds, blueberries, and a dash of cinnamon.
- **Lunch:**
- Quinoa and Black Bean Bowl: Mix cooked quinoa, black beans, corn, diced bell peppers, and a lime-cilantro dressing.

- **Dinner:**
- Grilled Veggie Stir-Fry: Combine a variety of colorful vegetables with tofu or lean protein. Serve over brown rice.

Day 11

- **Breakfast:**
- Whole Wheat Toast with Avocado: Spread avocado on whole wheat toast and sprinkle with red pepper flakes.
- **Lunch:**
- Lentil and Vegetable Soup: Prepare a hearty soup with lentils, carrots, celery, onions, and low-sodium vegetable broth.
- **Dinner:**
- Lemon Herb Roasted Chicken: Pair with roasted sweet potatoes and steamed asparagus.

Day 12

- **Breakfast:**
- Smoothie Bowl: Blend frozen banana, spinach, almond milk, and a scoop of protein powder. Top with sliced almonds and fresh fruit.

- **Lunch:**
- Tuna Salad Lettuce Wraps: Mix canned tuna, diced celery, red onion, and light mayo. Wrap in lettuce leaves.
- **Dinner:**
- Grilled Vegetable and Quinoa Stuffed Bell Peppers: Serve with a side salad.

Day 13

- **Breakfast:**
- Scrambled Eggs with Veggies: Sauté bell peppers, onions, and spinach. Mix with scrambled eggs and a sprinkle of low-fat cheese.
- **Lunch:**
- Hummus and Veggie Wrap: Spread hummus on a whole wheat tortilla, add sliced cucumber, shredded carrots, and baby spinach.
- **Dinner:**
- Baked Cod: Serve with roasted Brussels sprouts and a quinoa salad with cherry tomatoes and parsley.

Day 14

- **Breakfast:**
- Chia Seed Pudding: Combine chia seeds, almond milk, vanilla extract, and a touch of honey.

Refrigerate overnight and top with mixed berries.

- **Lunch:**
- Roasted Vegetable Quinoa Bowl: Mix roasted vegetables, cooked quinoa, and a drizzle of balsamic vinaigrette.
- **Dinner:**
- Grilled Portobello Mushrooms: Serve as "burgers" on whole wheat buns, with a side of grilled zucchini.

Feel free to continue the cycle of delicious and heart-healthy meals, incorporating a variety of fruits, vegetables, lean proteins, whole grains, and healthy fats. Rotate different sources of protein, experiment with various vegetables, and adjust portion sizes to match your activity level and personal requirements.

Remember, staying hydrated is essential throughout this meal plan. Opt for water, herbal teas, and limit caffeine and alcohol intake.

Additionally, consider snacking on nuts, seeds, fruits, and raw vegetables between meals to keep your energy levels steady.

CHAPTER THREE

Afib Diet Breakfast Recipes

1. Berry and Spinach Smoothie

Ingredients:

- 1 cup spinach leaves
- 1/2 cup mixed berries (blueberries, strawberries, raspberries)
- 1 small banana
- 1 tablespoon chia seeds
- 1 scoop protein powder (optional)
- 1 cup almond milk or any preferred milk

Instructions:

1. In a blender, combine spinach, mixed berries, banana, chia seeds, protein powder (if using), and almond milk.

2. Blend on high until smooth and creamy.

3. Pour into a glass and enjoy immediately.

Cooking Time: 5 minutes

2. Greek Yogurt Parfait

Ingredients:

- 1 cup Greek yogurt
- 1/4 cup granola (low-sugar)
- 1/2 cup mixed berries (strawberries, blueberries, raspberries)
- 1 teaspoon honey (optional)

Instructions:

1. In a glass or bowl, layer Greek yogurt, granola, and mixed berries.

2. Drizzle with honey if desired.

3. Repeat the layers and finish with a sprinkle of granola on top.

Cooking Time: 5 minutes

3. Oatmeal with Almonds and Berries

Ingredients:

- 1/2 cup rolled oats
- 1 cup water or milk of choice

- 1/4 cup sliced almonds

- 1/4 cup mixed berries (blueberries, raspberries)

- 1/2 teaspoon cinnamon

- 1 teaspoon honey (optional)

Instructions:

1. In a saucepan, bring water or milk to a boil.

2. Add rolled oats and cook according to package instructions.

3. Once cooked, stir in sliced almonds and cinnamon.

4. Top with mixed berries and drizzle with honey if desired.

Cooking Time: 10 minutes

4. Whole Wheat Toast with Avocado

Ingredients:

- 2 slices whole wheat bread, toasted

- 1 ripe avocado

- Red pepper flakes

- Salt and pepper to taste

Instructions:

1. Cut the avocado in half, remove the pit, and scoop the flesh into a bowl.

2. Mash the avocado with a fork and season with salt and pepper.

3. Spread the mashed avocado onto the toasted whole wheat bread slices.

4. Sprinkle with red pepper flakes for a kick of flavor.

Cooking Time: 5 minutes

5. Chia Seed Pudding

Ingredients:

- 3 tablespoons chia seeds
- 1 cup almond milk or any preferred milk
- 1/2 teaspoon vanilla extract
- 1 teaspoon honey or maple syrup
- Fresh fruit for topping (e.g., sliced strawberries, kiwi, banana)

Instructions:

1. In a bowl, mix chia seeds, almond milk, vanilla extract, and honey/maple syrup.

2. Stir well to ensure the chia seeds are evenly distributed.

3. Cover and refrigerate for at least 2 hours or overnight, allowing the chia seeds to absorb the liquid and thicken.

4. When ready to eat, give the pudding a good stir and top with fresh fruit.

Cooking Time: 5 minutes (plus chilling time)

Afib Diet Lunch Recipes

1. Grilled Chicken Salad

Ingredients:

- 4 oz grilled chicken breast, sliced
- 2 cups mixed greens (spinach, lettuce, arugula)
- 1/2 cucumber, sliced
- 1/2 bell pepper, diced
- 1/4 cup cherry tomatoes, halved
- Light vinaigrette dressing

Instructions:

1. Arrange mixed greens on a plate.

2. Top with sliced grilled chicken, cucumber, bell pepper, and cherry tomatoes.

3. Drizzle with a light vinaigrette dressing.

Cooking Time: 15 minutes (if chicken is pre-cooked)

2. Chickpea and Avocado Salad

Ingredients:

- 1 can (15 oz) chickpeas, drained and rinsed
- 1 avocado, diced
- 1/4 red onion, finely chopped
- Fresh cilantro, chopped
- Juice of 1 lime
- Feta cheese (optional)
- Salt and pepper to taste

Instructions:

1. In a bowl, combine chickpeas, diced avocado, red onion, and cilantro.

2. Squeeze lime juice over the mixture and gently toss to combine.

3. Add salt and pepper to taste, and sprinkle with feta cheese if desired.

Cooking Time: 10 minutes

3. Lentil and Vegetable Soup

Ingredients:

- 1 cup cooked green or brown lentils
- 2 carrots, diced
- 2 celery stalks, diced
- 1 onion, chopped
- 2 cloves garlic, minced
- 4 cups low-sodium vegetable broth
- 1 teaspoon dried thyme
- Salt and pepper to taste

Instructions:

1. In a pot, sauté onion and garlic until fragrant.

2. Add carrots and celery, and cook for a few minutes.

3. Stir in cooked lentils, vegetable broth, dried thyme, salt, and pepper.

4. Simmer for about 20 minutes until vegetables are tender.

5. Serve warm as a hearty and nutritious lunch.

Cooking Time: 30 minutes

4. Tuna Salad Lettuce Wraps

Ingredients:

- 1 can (5 oz) tuna, drained
- 1/4 cup diced celery
- 1/4 red onion, finely chopped
- Light mayo or Greek yogurt (to taste)
- Lettuce leaves (such as Romaine or Bibb)

Instructions:

1. In a bowl, combine tuna, diced celery, and chopped red onion.
2. Add light mayo or Greek yogurt and mix until well combined.
3. Spoon the tuna salad into lettuce leaves and wrap them up.

Cooking Time: 10 minutes

5. Quinoa and Black Bean Bowl

Ingredients:

- 1 cup cooked quinoa
- 1 can (15 oz) black beans, drained and rinsed
- 1/2 cup corn kernels (fresh, frozen, or canned)
- 1/2 red bell pepper, diced
- Lime-cilantro dressing

Instructions:

1. In a bowl, combine cooked quinoa, black beans, corn, and diced red bell pepper.

2. Drizzle with lime-cilantro dressing and toss to combine.

Cooking Time: 15 minutes (if quinoa is pre-cooked)

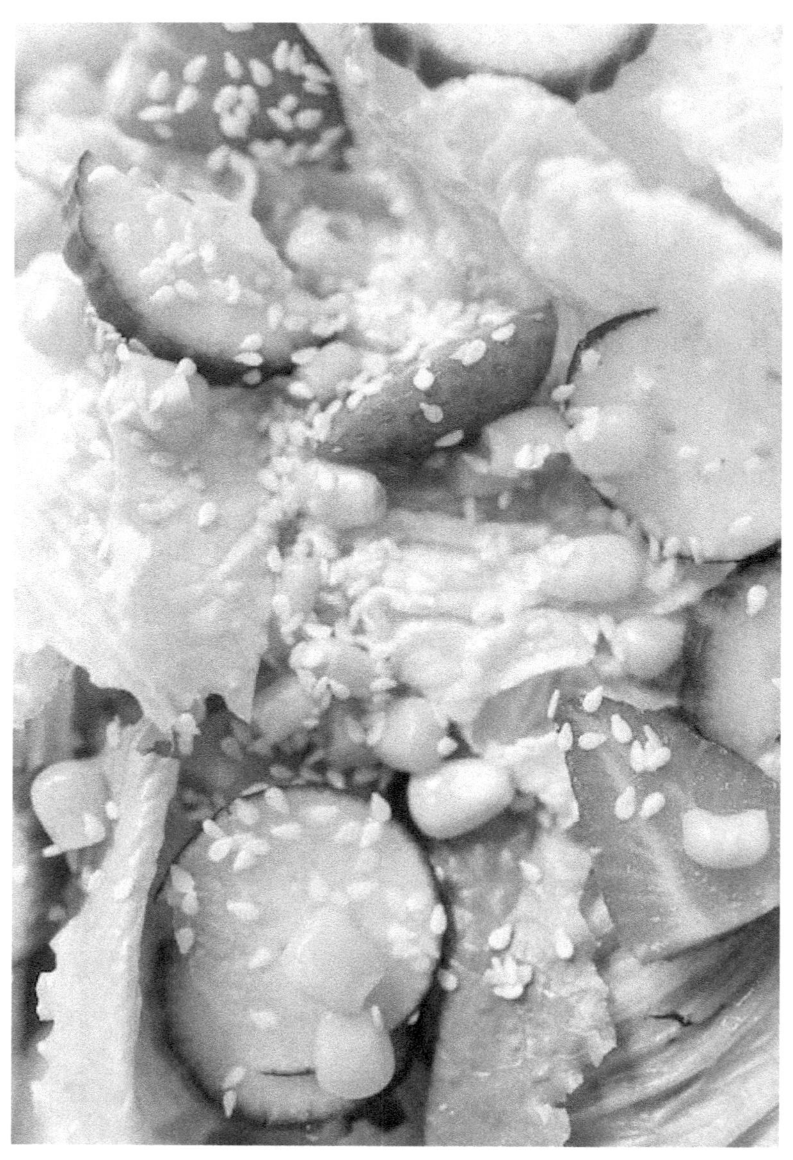

CHAPTER FOUR

Afib Diet Dinner Recipes

1. Baked Salmon with Quinoa and Broccoli

Ingredients:

- 6 oz salmon fillet
- 1/2 cup cooked quinoa
- 1 cup broccoli florets
- Lemon juice
- Olive oil
- Dill (fresh or dried)
- Salt and pepper to taste

Instructions:

1. Preheat the oven to 375°F (190°C).

2. Place the salmon on a baking sheet and drizzle with lemon juice and a touch of olive oil.

3. Sprinkle dill, salt, and pepper over the salmon.

4. Arrange broccoli florets around the salmon on the baking sheet.

5. Bake for about 15-20 minutes or until the salmon is cooked through and flakes easily.

6. Serve the baked salmon with cooked quinoa and steamed broccoli.

Cooking Time: 20-25 minutes

2. Turkey Meatballs with Whole Wheat Pasta

Ingredients:

- 4-6 turkey meatballs (pre-made or homemade)
- 1 cup whole wheat pasta (cooked)
- Tomato sauce (low-sodium and no added sugar)
- Grated Parmesan cheese (optional)

Instructions:

1. Heat the turkey meatballs in a skillet or oven according to package instructions.
2. Warm the tomato sauce in a separate pot.
3. Serve the turkey meatballs over cooked whole wheat pasta and top with tomato sauce.
4. Sprinkle with grated Parmesan cheese if desired.

Cooking Time: Varies based on meatball type (usually 15-20 minutes)

3. Grilled Vegetable Stir-Fry

Ingredients:

- Assorted vegetables (bell peppers, zucchini, carrots, onions, mushrooms, etc.), sliced
- Tofu or lean protein (chicken, shrimp, or tempeh)
- Low-sodium soy sauce
- Garlic and ginger (minced)
- Olive oil
- Brown rice (cooked)

Instructions:

1. Heat olive oil in a pan or wok over medium-high heat.

2. Add minced garlic and ginger, and sauté until fragrant.

3. Add sliced vegetables and tofu or protein of choice.

4. Stir-fry until vegetables are tender and protein is cooked.

5. Drizzle with low-sodium soy sauce and continue to cook briefly.

6. Serve over cooked brown rice.

Cooking Time: 20-25 minutes

4. Lemon Herb Roasted Chicken with Sweet Potatoes

Ingredients:

- 4 oz boneless, skinless chicken breast
- 1 medium sweet potato, peeled and cubed
- Lemon zest and juice
- Fresh herbs (rosemary, thyme)
- Olive oil
- Salt and pepper to taste

Instructions:

1. Preheat the oven to 400°F (200°C).

2. In a bowl, mix lemon zest, lemon juice, chopped fresh herbs, olive oil, salt, and pepper.

3. Coat the chicken breast with the marinade and let it sit for a few minutes.

4. Place the marinated chicken and cubed sweet potatoes on a baking sheet.

5. Roast in the oven for about 20-25 minutes or until the chicken is cooked through and sweet potatoes are tender.

Cooking Time: 25-30 minutes

5. Grilled Portobello Mushroom Burgers

Ingredients:

- 2 large Portobello mushroom caps
- Whole wheat burger buns
- Marinade (balsamic vinegar, olive oil, garlic, herbs)
- Toppings: lettuce, tomato, onion, avocado
- Cheese (optional)

Instructions:

1. In a bowl, mix balsamic vinegar, olive oil, minced garlic, and your choice of herbs.

2. Brush the Portobello mushroom caps with the marinade.

3. Grill the mushroom caps on medium heat for about 5-7 minutes on each side.

4. Toast the whole wheat burger buns on the grill.

5. Assemble the mushroom burgers with lettuce, tomato, onion, avocado, and cheese (if desired).

Cooking Time: 15-20 minutes

Afib Diet Dessert Recipes

1. Mixed Berry Parfait

Ingredients:

- 1 cup mixed berries (blueberries, raspberries, strawberries)
- 1 cup Greek yogurt (plain, non-fat)
- 1 tablespoon honey or maple syrup
- 1/4 cup granola (low-sugar)

Instructions:

1. In a glass or bowl, layer Greek yogurt, mixed berries, and granola.

2. Drizzle honey or maple syrup over the layers.

3. Repeat the layers and finish with a sprinkle of granola on top.

Cooking Time: 10 minutes

2. Dark Chocolate-Dipped Strawberries

Ingredients:

- Fresh strawberries (as many as desired)
- Dark chocolate chips (70% cocoa or higher)

Instructions:

1. Wash and dry the strawberries, leaving the stems intact.

2. Melt the dark chocolate in a microwave-safe bowl in 20-second intervals, stirring in between until smooth.

3. Dip each strawberry into the melted chocolate, letting any excess drip off.

4. Place the dipped strawberries on a parchment paper-lined tray.

5. Allow the chocolate to set by refrigerating the strawberries for about 30 minutes.

Cooking Time: 20 minutes (plus chilling time)

3. Banana Oat Cookies

Ingredients:

- 2 ripe bananas, mashed
- 1 cup rolled oats
- 1/4 cup chopped nuts (walnuts, almonds)
- 1/4 cup dark chocolate chips (optional)
- 1/2 teaspoon vanilla extract
- Pinch of cinnamon

Instructions:

1. Preheat the oven to 350°F (175°C).

2. In a bowl, mix mashed bananas, rolled oats, chopped nuts, dark chocolate chips (if using), vanilla extract, and cinnamon.

3. Drop spoonfuls of the mixture onto a baking sheet lined with parchment paper.

4. Flatten each spoonful slightly to form cookies.

5. Bake for about 15-20 minutes or until the cookies are golden and firm.

Cooking Time: 15-20 minutes

4. Chia Seed Pudding with Berries

Ingredients:

- 3 tablespoons chia seeds
- 1 cup almond milk or any preferred milk
- 1/2 teaspoon vanilla extract
- 1 teaspoon honey or maple syrup
- Mixed berries for topping (blueberries, raspberries, strawberries)

Instructions:

1. In a bowl, mix chia seeds, almond milk, vanilla extract, and honey/maple syrup.

2. Stir well to ensure the chia seeds are evenly distributed.

3. Cover and refrigerate for at least 2 hours or overnight, allowing the chia seeds to absorb the liquid and thicken.

4. When ready to serve, give the pudding a good stir and top with mixed berries.

Cooking Time: 5 minutes (plus chilling time)

5. Baked Apple with Cinnamon

Ingredients:

- 1 apple (Honeycrisp, Granny Smith)
- 1 teaspoon honey or maple syrup
- Ground cinnamon
- Chopped nuts (walnuts, almonds) for topping

Instructions:

1. Preheat the oven to 375°F (190°C).

2. Core the apple and place it in a baking dish.

3. Drizzle honey or maple syrup over the apple.

4. Sprinkle ground cinnamon over the apple, filling the core cavity as well.

5. Bake for about 20-25 minutes or until the apple is tender.

6. Remove from the oven and top with chopped nuts.

Cooking Time: 20-25 minutes

CHAPTER FIVE

Afib Diet Snacks Recipes

1. Nut Butter and Apple Slices

Ingredients:

- 1 medium apple, sliced
- 2 tablespoons nut butter (almond, peanut, or cashew)

Instructions:

1. Wash and slice the apple into thin rounds.

2. Spread a thin layer of nut butter on each apple slice.

3. Arrange the slices on a plate and enjoy the crisp and creamy combination.

2. Greek Yogurt with Berries

Ingredients:

- 1/2 cup Greek yogurt (plain, non-fat)
- 1/4 cup mixed berries (blueberries, raspberries, strawberries)

Instructions:

1. Spoon the Greek yogurt into a bowl.

2. Top with mixed berries for a burst of antioxidants and natural sweetness.

3. Mix gently or enjoy the layers separately.

3. Veggie Sticks with Hummus

Ingredients:

- Assorted vegetable sticks (carrots, celery, bell peppers, cucumber)
- Hummus (store-bought or homemade)

Instructions:

1. Wash, peel, and cut vegetables into sticks.

2. Serve with a side of hummus for dipping, providing a satisfying crunch and creaminess.

4. Roasted Chickpeas

Ingredients:

- 1 can (15 oz) chickpeas, drained and rinsed
- 1 tablespoon olive oil
- Spices (paprika, cumin, garlic powder, cayenne pepper)
- Salt and pepper to taste

Instructions:

1. Preheat the oven to 400°F (200°C).

2. In a bowl, toss chickpeas with olive oil and spices.

3. Spread the chickpeas on a baking sheet and roast for about 20-25 minutes, stirring occasionally.

4. Allow the chickpeas to cool before snacking on the crispy, flavorful bites.

5. Rice Cake with Avocado

Ingredients:

- 1 rice cake (whole grain)
- 1/4 ripe avocado

- Red pepper flakes (optional)
- Salt and pepper to taste

Instructions:

1. Spread the ripe avocado onto the rice cake.

2. Sprinkle with red pepper flakes for a touch of heat, and season with salt and pepper.

3. Enjoy the satisfying texture and flavors of this simple snack.

Afib Diet Juicing and Smoothies Recipes

1. Berry Antioxidant Smoothie

Ingredients:

- 1 cup mixed berries (blueberries, raspberries, strawberries)
- 1/2 banana
- 1 cup spinach leaves
- 1/2 cup Greek yogurt (plain, non-fat)
- 1/2 cup almond milk
- 1 tablespoon chia seeds

Instructions:

1. Combine mixed berries, banana, spinach, Greek yogurt, almond milk, and chia seeds in a blender.

2. Blend on high until smooth and creamy.

3. Pour into a glass and enjoy the antioxidant-rich goodness.

2. Green Detox Juice

Ingredients:

- 1 cucumber
- 2 celery stalks
- 1 green apple
- Handful of kale or spinach
- 1/2 lemon (peeled)
- 1-inch piece of ginger (peeled)

Instructions:

1. Wash and prep the cucumber, celery, apple, kale or spinach, lemon, and ginger.

2. Run all the ingredients through a juicer.

3. Stir the juice well and serve immediately for a refreshing green detox.

3. Heart-Healthy Beet Smoothie

Ingredients:

- 1 small cooked beet, peeled and chopped
- 1/2 cup mixed berries (blueberries, strawberries)
- 1/4 cup Greek yogurt (plain, non-fat)
- 1 tablespoon flaxseeds
- 1/2 cup almond milk
- Honey or maple syrup to taste

Instructions:

1. Blend cooked beet, mixed berries, Greek yogurt, flaxseeds, almond milk, and sweetener (if desired) in a blender.

2. Blend until smooth and vibrant.

3. Pour into a glass and enjoy the earthy-sweet goodness.

4. Citrus Energy Booster Juice

Ingredients:

- 2 oranges, peeled
- 1 grapefruit, peeled
- 1 small carrot

- 1/2 lemon (peeled)
- 1-inch piece of turmeric (optional)
- Pinch of cayenne pepper (optional)

Instructions:

1. Prepare the oranges, grapefruit, carrot, lemon, and turmeric.

2. Run all the ingredients through a juicer.

3. Stir well and add a pinch of cayenne pepper for a zesty kick.

5. Creamy Avocado Banana Smoothie

Ingredients:

- 1/2 ripe avocado
- 1 banana
- 1 cup spinach or kale
- 1 cup almond milk
- 1 tablespoon almond butter
- 1 teaspoon honey or maple syrup

Instructions:

1. Blend ripe avocado, banana, spinach or kale, almond milk, almond butter, and sweetener in a blender.

2. Blend until smooth and creamy.

3. Pour into a glass and enjoy the creamy and satisfying blend.

Cooking Time: Most smoothies and juices take about 5 minutes to prepare, with variations based on ingredients and equipment used.

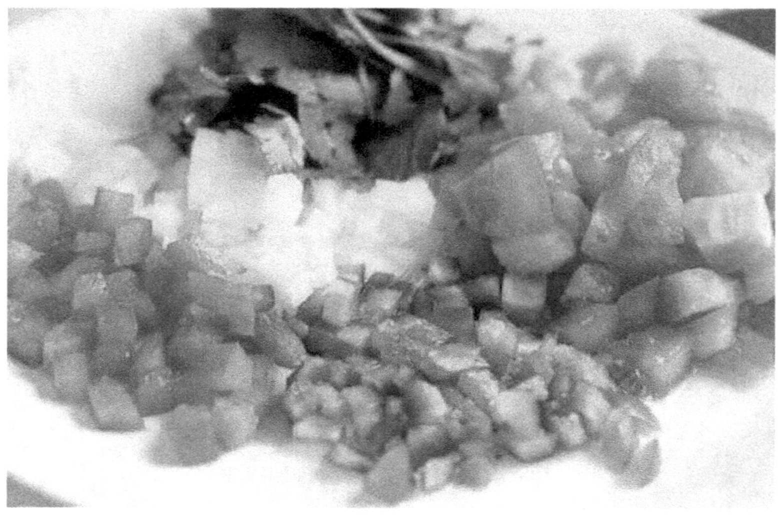

CONCLUSION

In conclusion, the AFib diet stands as a powerful ally in the journey towards managing atrial fibrillation and promoting overall heart health. This dietary approach, centered around nutrient-rich foods and mindful eating, offers a myriad of benefits that extend far beyond the confines of managing a specific condition.

By focusing on whole foods like fruits, vegetables, lean proteins, whole grains, and healthy fats, individuals with AFib can provide their bodies with a comprehensive array of vitamins, minerals, antioxidants, and essential nutrients.

These elements collectively contribute to reducing inflammation, stabilizing blood pressure, and supporting cardiovascular function, which are all essential factors for managing atrial fibrillation.

The benefits of the AFib diet extend beyond the confines of the heart alone. By adopting this approach, individuals may find themselves shedding excess weight or maintaining a healthy weight, thus reducing the strain on the cardiovascular system and improving overall heart function.

Additionally, the emphasis on nutrient-dense foods provides a sustained energy source, reducing feelings of fatigue and enhancing the ability to engage in physical activity.

One of the most significant advantages of the AFib diet is its potential to empower individuals to take an active role in their health management.

Through making informed food choices, individuals can exert a degree of control over their condition, potentially reducing the frequency and severity of AFib episodes. However, it is crucial to remember that while the AFib diet can be highly beneficial, it is not a standalone solution.

Collaborating closely with healthcare professionals, such as cardiologists and dietitians, is essential to tailor the diet to individual needs and ensure that it complements any medical treatment or medication that may be necessary.

The diverse array of recipes provided, from hearty breakfasts to delectable desserts, illustrates the versatility of the AFib diet. Whether it's enjoying a nutrient-packed smoothie in the morning, indulging in a nourishing lunch, or savoring a heart-healthy dinner, the AFib diet can be both fulfilling and satisfying.

These recipes also underscore the importance of balance, showing that deliciousness and healthiness are not mutually exclusive.

In essence, the AFib diet presents a holistic approach to managing atrial fibrillation. Beyond the physical health benefits, it advocates for mindful eating, encouraging individuals to be more attuned to their body's needs and the impact of their food choices.

This approach can cultivate a greater sense of well-being, as individuals connect with their bodies and engage in a lifestyle that supports long-term health.

As we've explored the principles, benefits, and practical aspects of the AFib diet, it becomes evident that this dietary approach is more than just a means to an end—it's a path to better living. Armed with knowledge and guided by medical professionals, individuals can embark on this journey to embrace an AFib diet that is tailored to their unique needs, preferences, and health goals.

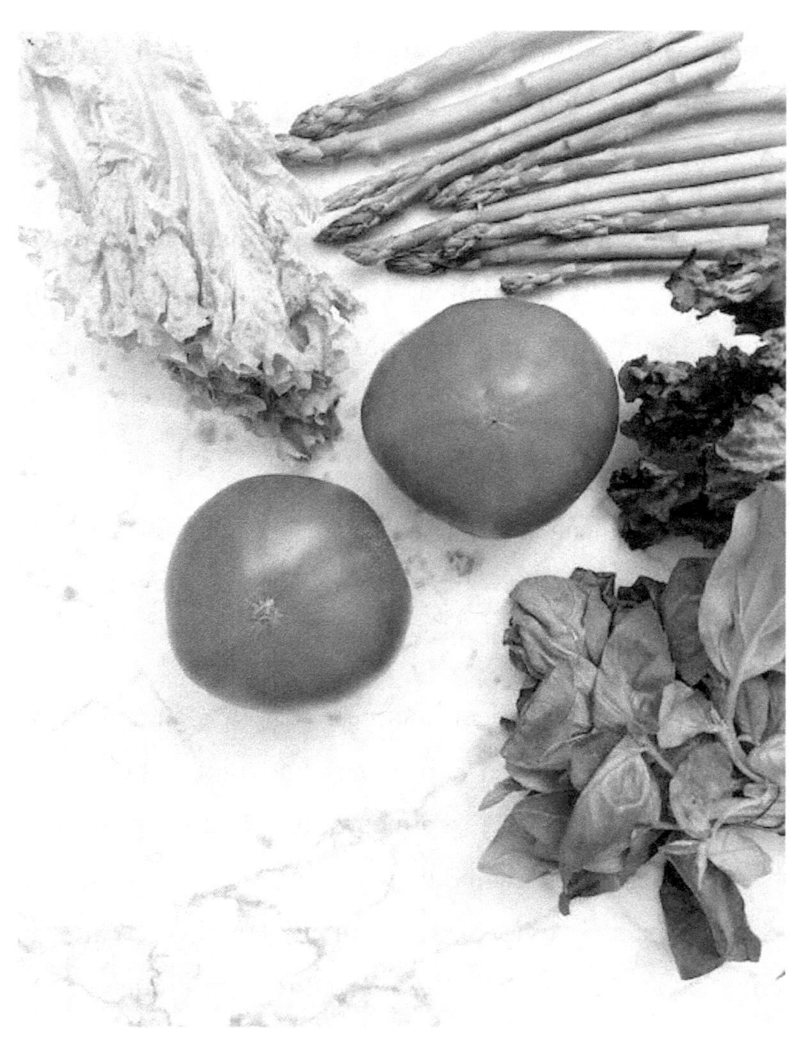